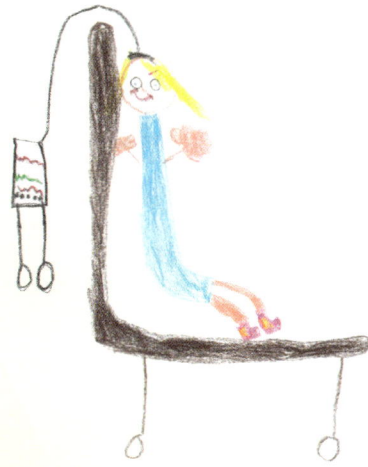

The Girl Who Had a

Big Adventure

Cancer, Chemo & Cupcakes

STACIA MERS & JANE FREUND

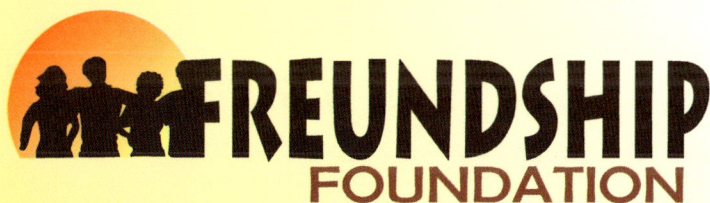

FREUNDSHIP
FOUNDATION

Positively influencing lives through friendship, communication, and education.

ISBN-13: 978-0-9839957-3-9

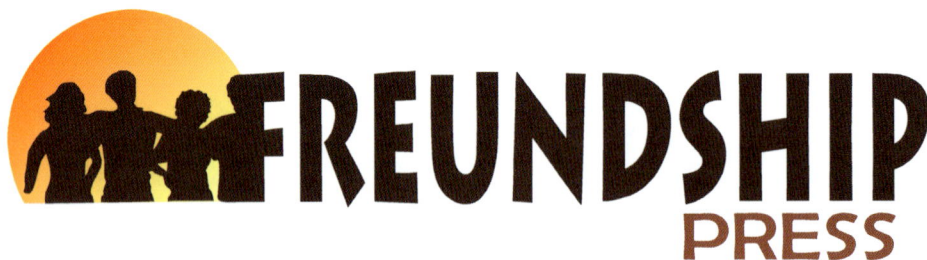

FREUNDSHIP
PRESS

Positively influencing lives through friendship, communication, and education.

PO Box 9171 • Boise, ID 83707 • (208) 407-7457
www.freundshippress.com • info@freundshippress.com

A portion of the proceeds from the sale of this book will be donated to non-profit organizations focused on childhood cancer research.

ACKNOWLEDGEMENTS

I want to thank St. Luke's Children's Hospital and MSTI Peds in Boise, ID for helping me get through my cancer treatment. I also want to thank Jane Freund for helping me tell my story which will hopefully help other kids going through what I went through. And last but not least, my family for supporting me. – **Stacia Mers, 8, brain cancer survivor**

Thank you to Stacia for allowing me the opportunity to tell her story which will help countless other children and their families as they face their own cancer battles. Also, thank you to the rest of the Mers family (Lori, Mike and Bryce) for showing how to support somebody through cancer whether as parents or siblings. I am amazingly blessed to have had the Mers' support through my own cancer journey. Finally, thank you to Thom Hollis of Hollis Design Studios for designing the cover and laying out the book. – **Jane Freund, more than 8, thyroid cancer survivor**

INTRODUCTION

Stacia - I wanted to write a book about my cancer because I wanted to tell kids what is going to happen when they have cancer. I also wanted not only my family and close friends to know what I went through, but I also wanted others to know, too. I hope you learn a bit about my cancer and enjoy my book!

Lori (Stacia's Mom) - Stacia was diagnosed at six years old with medulloblastoma - a form of brain cancer. Following her Kindergarten Valentine's Day Party in February 2010, she had an MRI which confirmed a tumor the size of a small lemon in the cerebellum (the back of the brain). This was the day her journey began, and she has been one little fighter since that very first day displaying much courage, strength and determination. As Stacia's Mom, I couldn't be more proud that she wanted to share her story about her cancer journey with others. She wanted to educate other young children - those who are just beginning their own journey as well as those who might know someone who has cancer but are unfamiliar with cancer and all that accompanies such a diagnosis.

As a mother of a young child with cancer, I searched for books and information for our entire family which might help us all maneuver this unfamiliar path. My search was less than stellar, which was much of the reason we encouraged Stacia to tell her story. She tells it in her words with her own pictures. Many thanks go out to Jane Freund (our family friend) who worked closely with Stacia to make this all possible! You rock, Stacia! I'm so very proud of you!

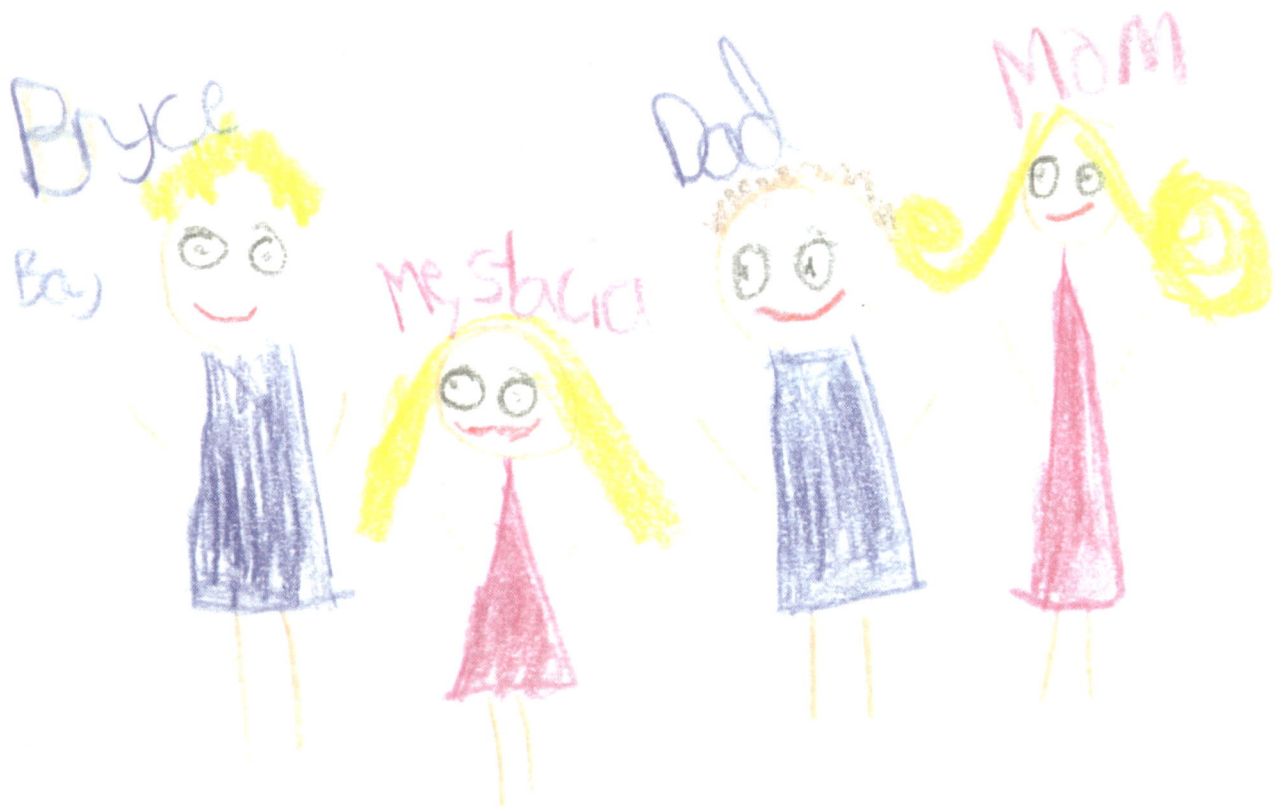

Bryce
Boy

mestacia

Dad

Mom

My Family

This is my family. I have a Mom and
Dad and an older brother named Bryce.
In this picture, I am in kindergarten.

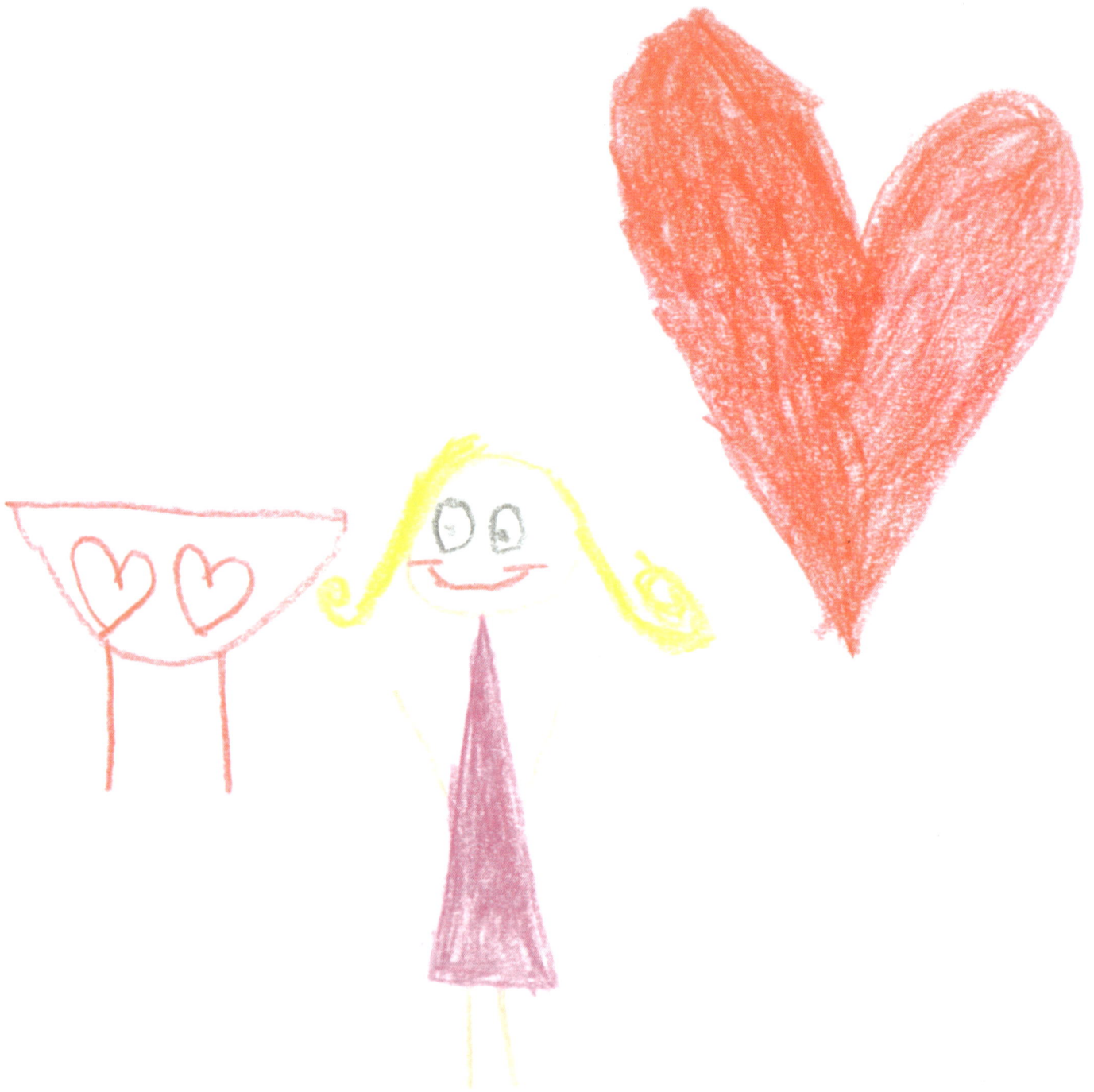

I went to my kindergarten Valentine's Day party and had a good time. After the party, I went to the doctor because I had double vision and headaches.

Exit

The doctor said I needed
to have an MRI that day.

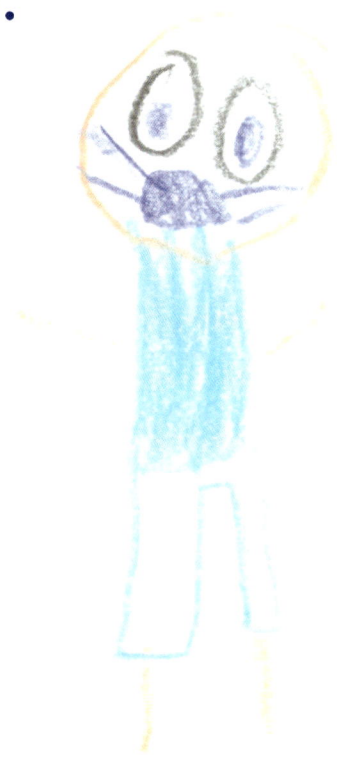

The MRI took a picture
of my brain.

3

That picture showed I had a brain
tumor, and it was probably cancer.
Mom, Dad, Bryce and I were all very sad!

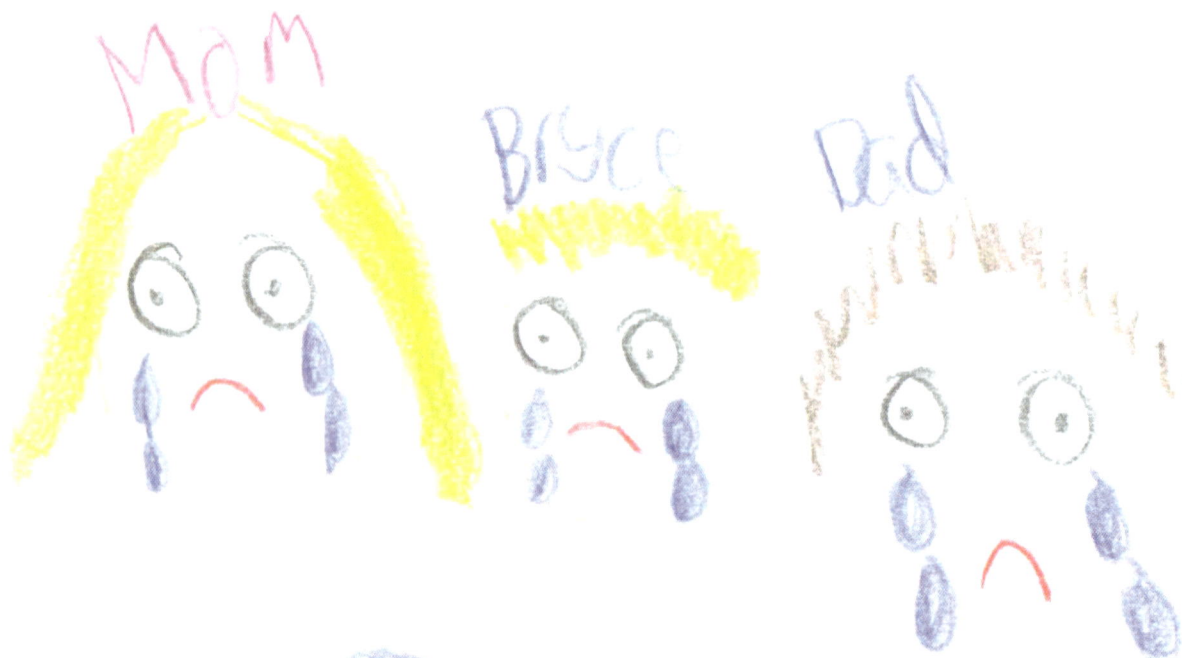

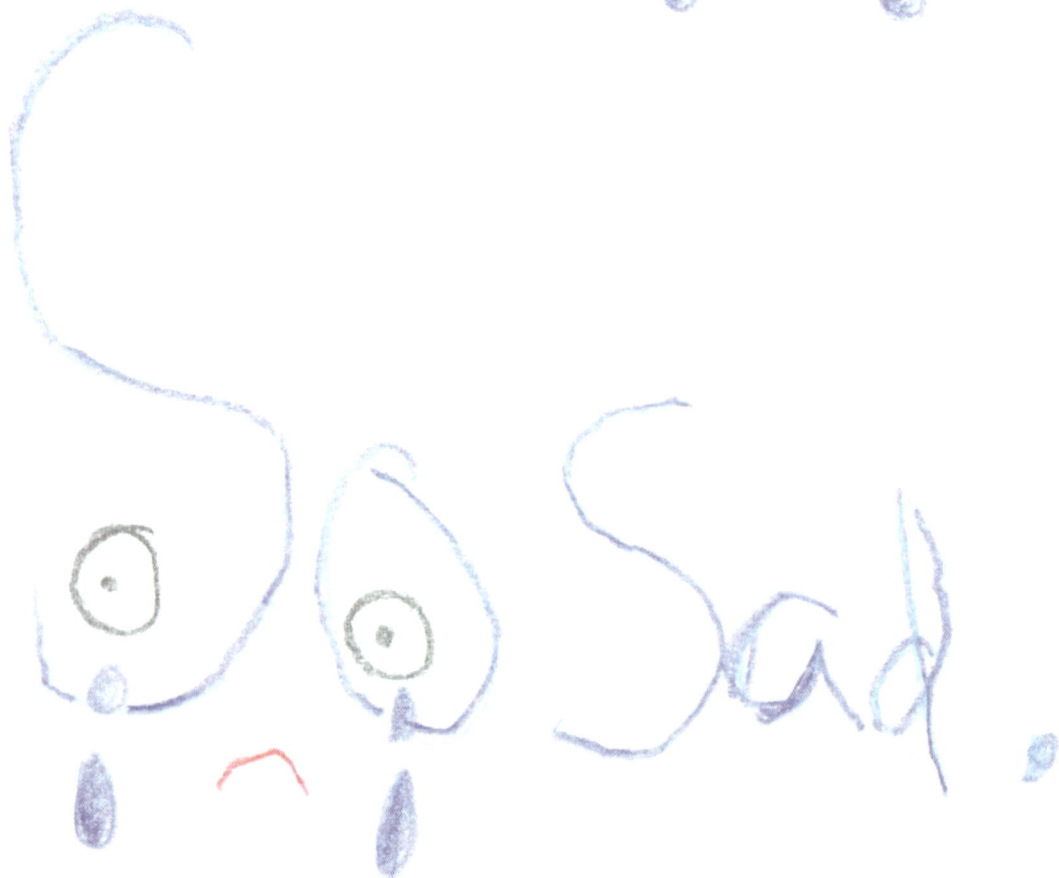

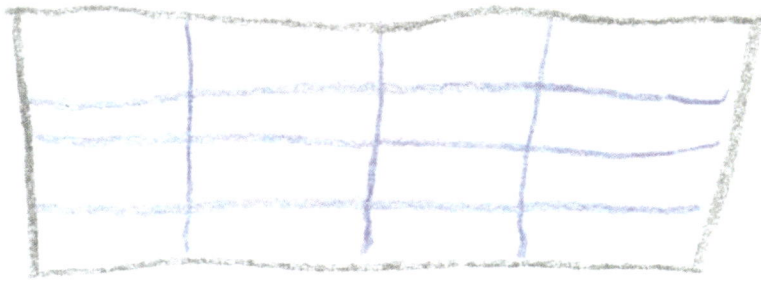

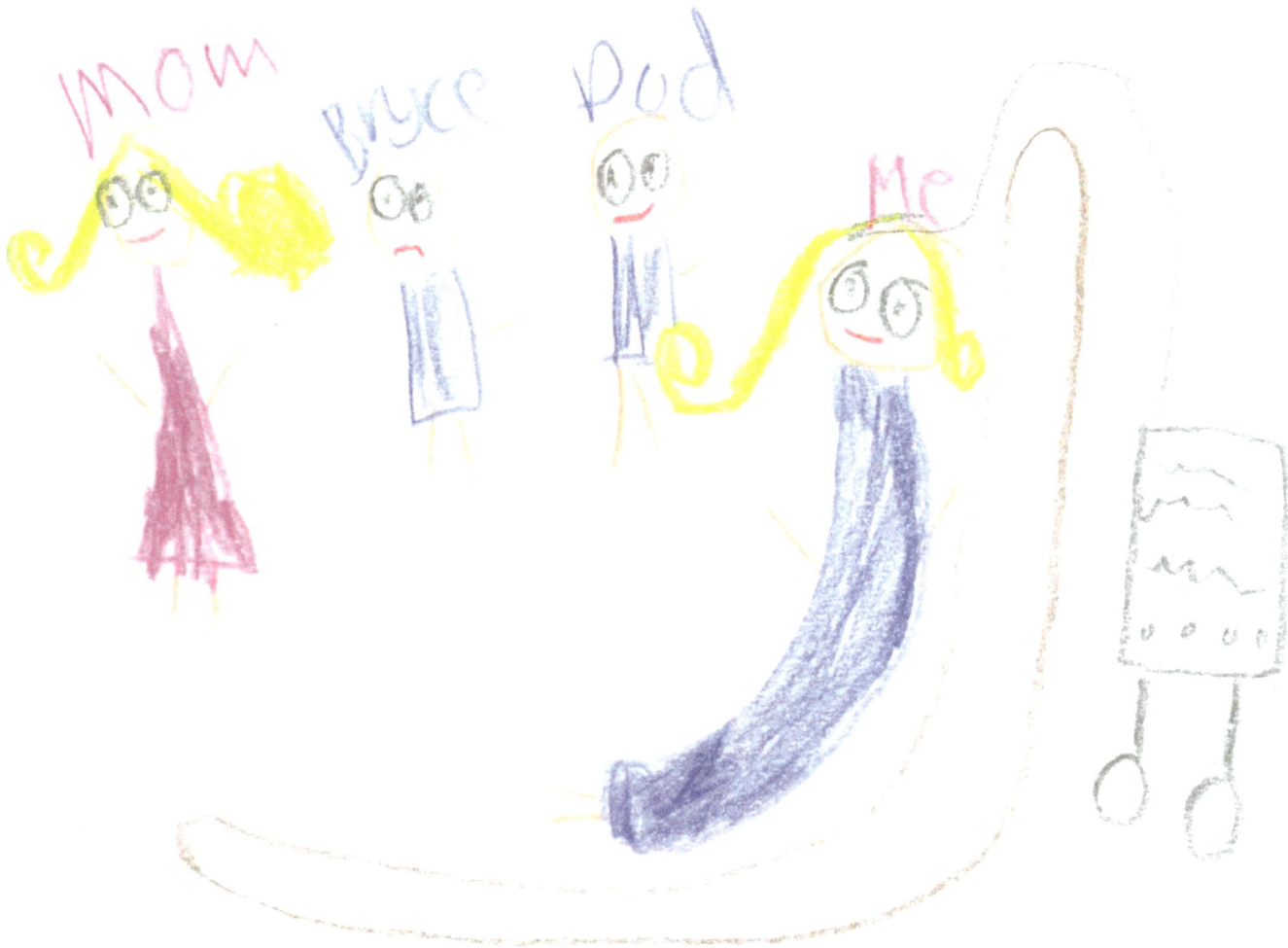

That night, I had to have a shunt put into my head to drain out the extra fluid. It was like I had an overflowing bathtub in my head, and the shunt pulled the plug.

The next day, Mom and I went in an ambulance to another hospital.

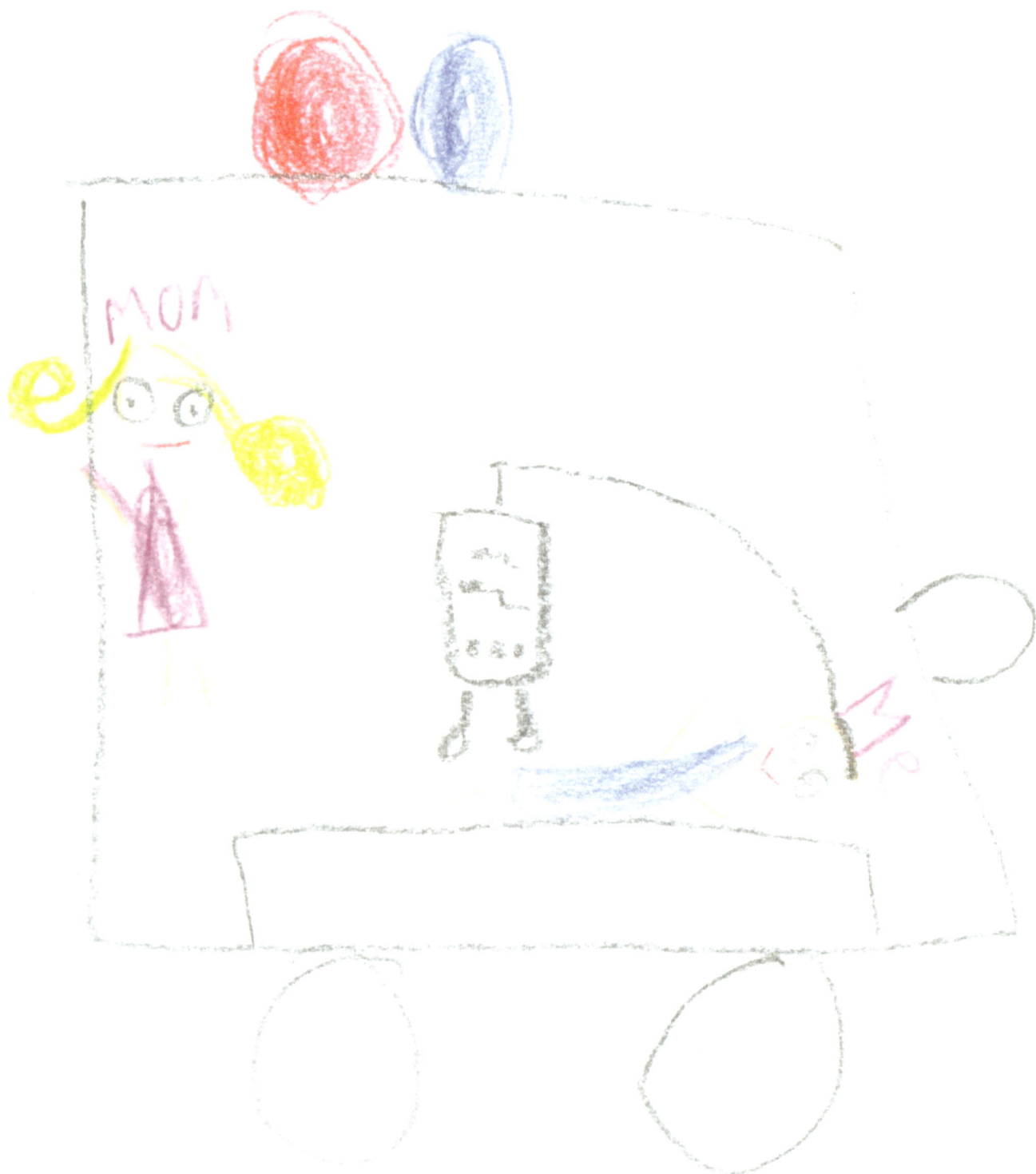

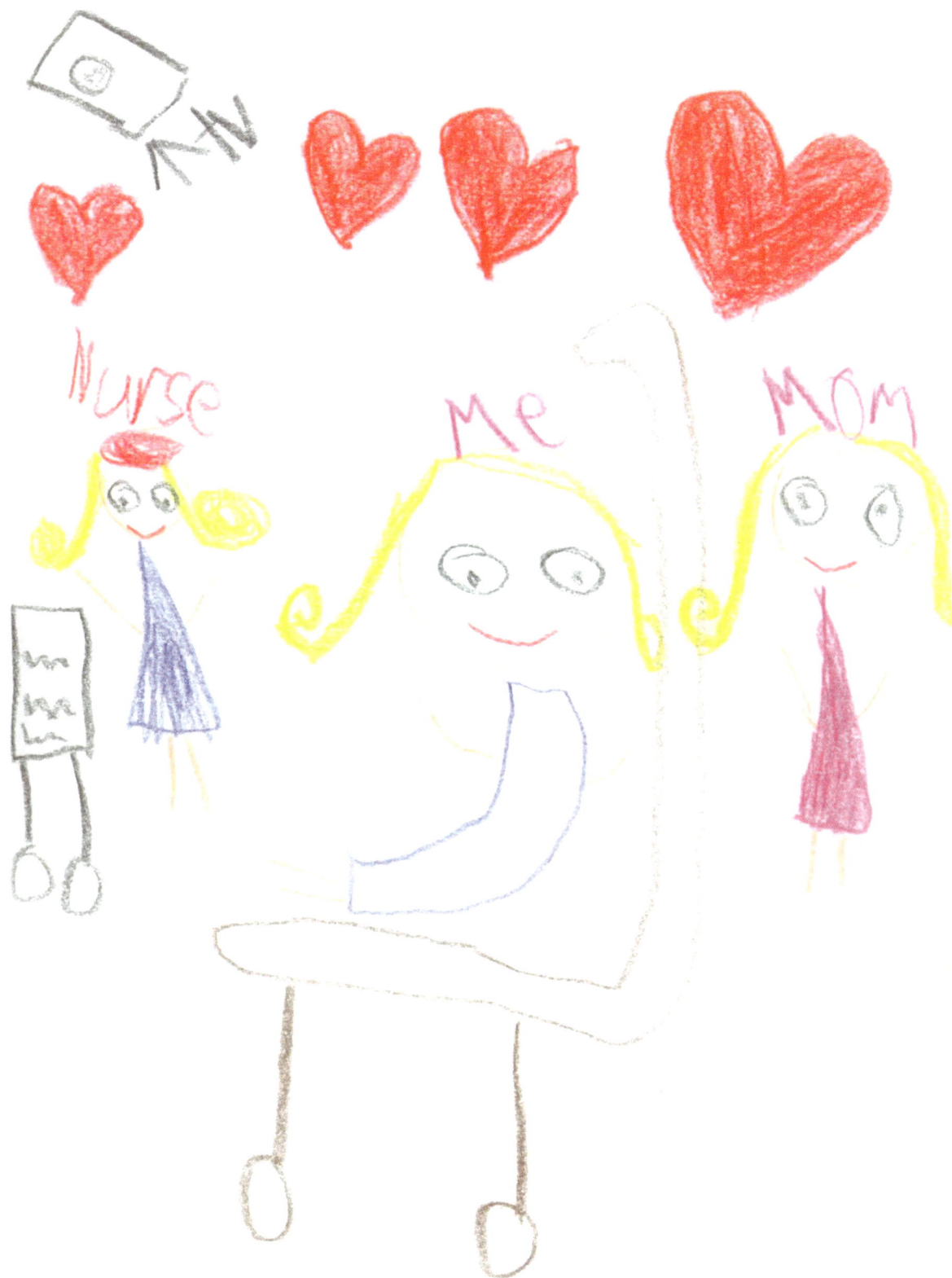

I had to wait three days to have my surgery. Mom and I made paper hearts because it was Valentine's Day.

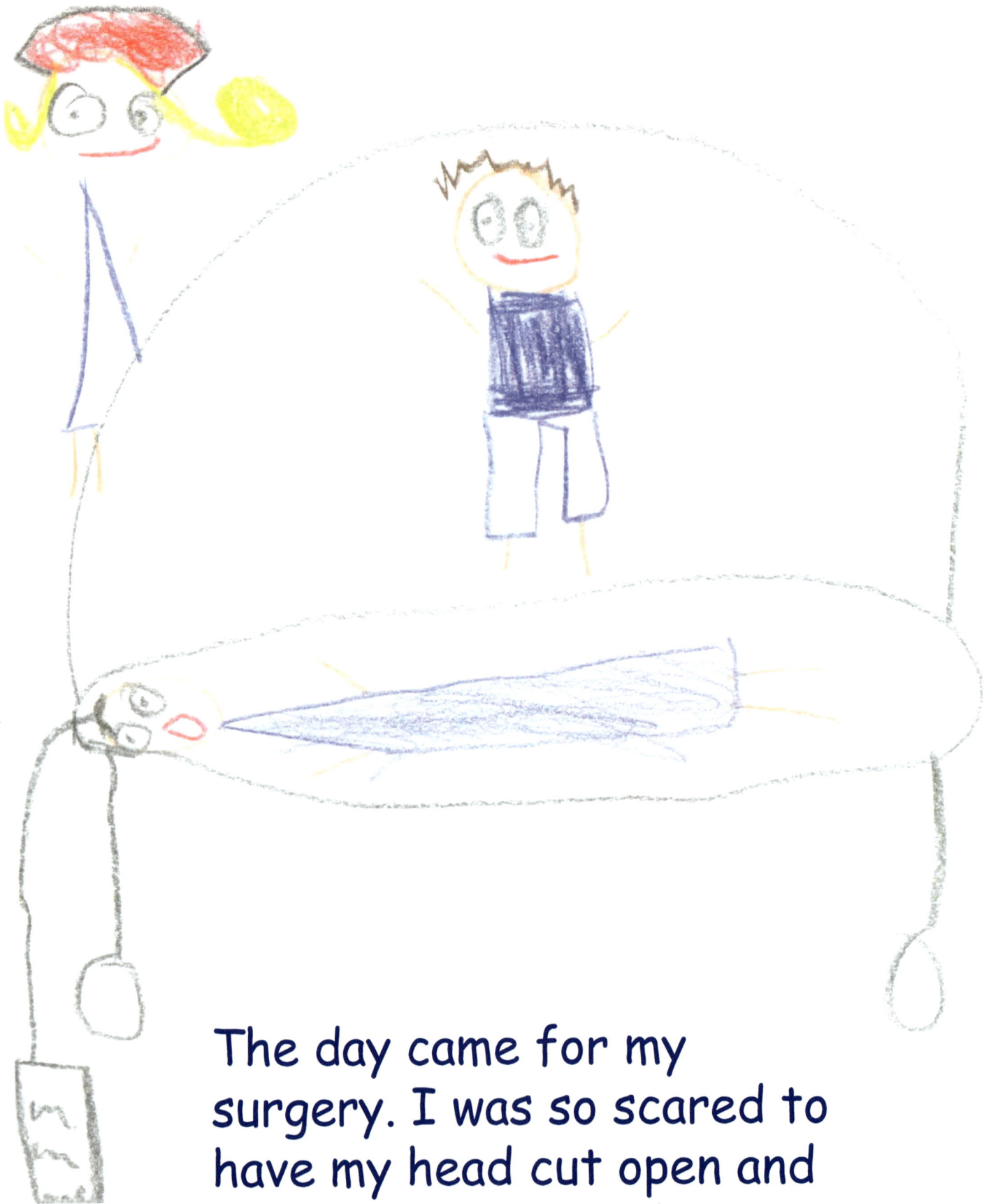

The day came for my surgery. I was so scared to have my head cut open and my tumor taken out!

All of the people were in the waiting room waiting to hear how my surgery turned out.

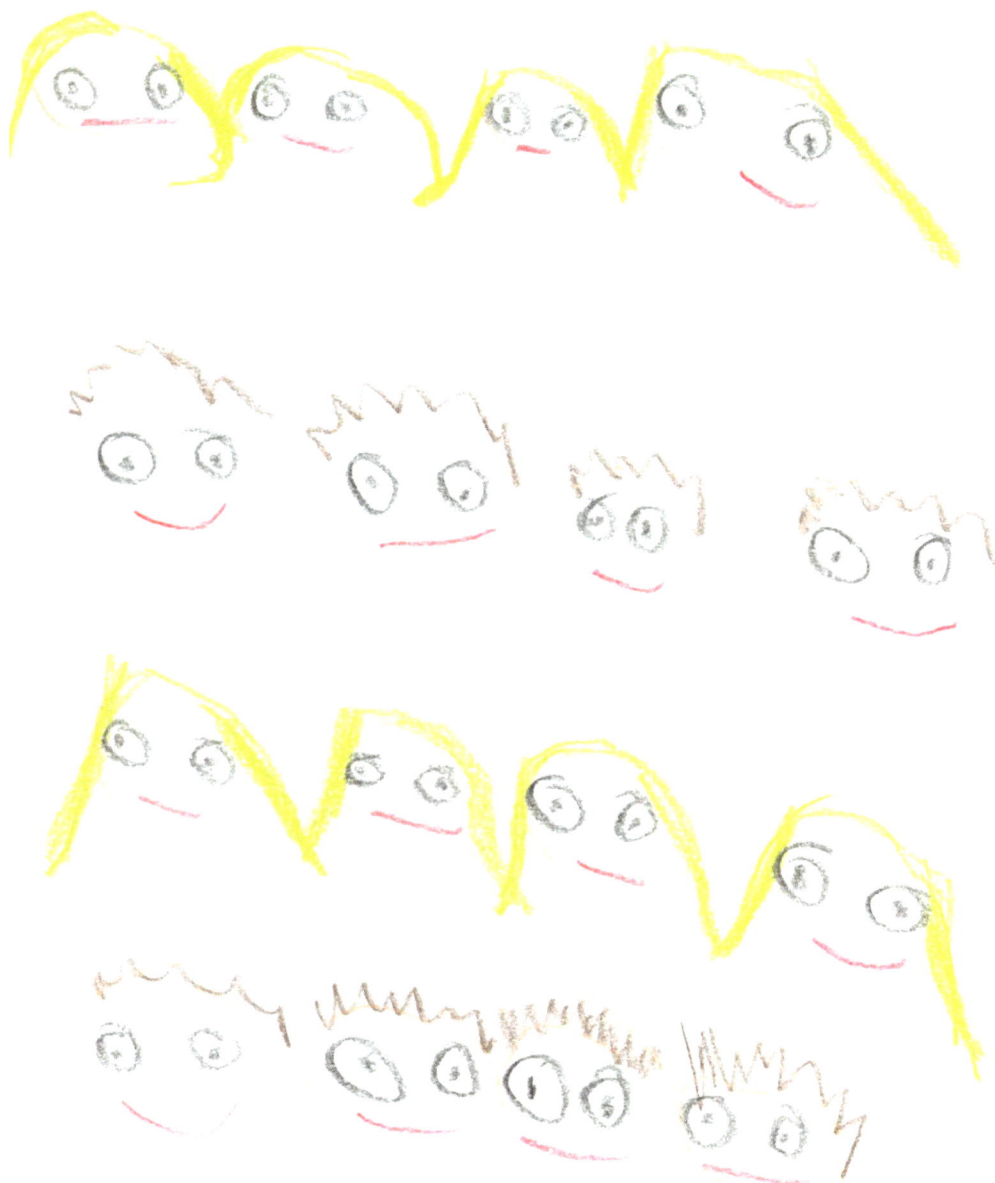

The surgery took eight hours, and the tumor was cancer. It was the size of a small lemon.

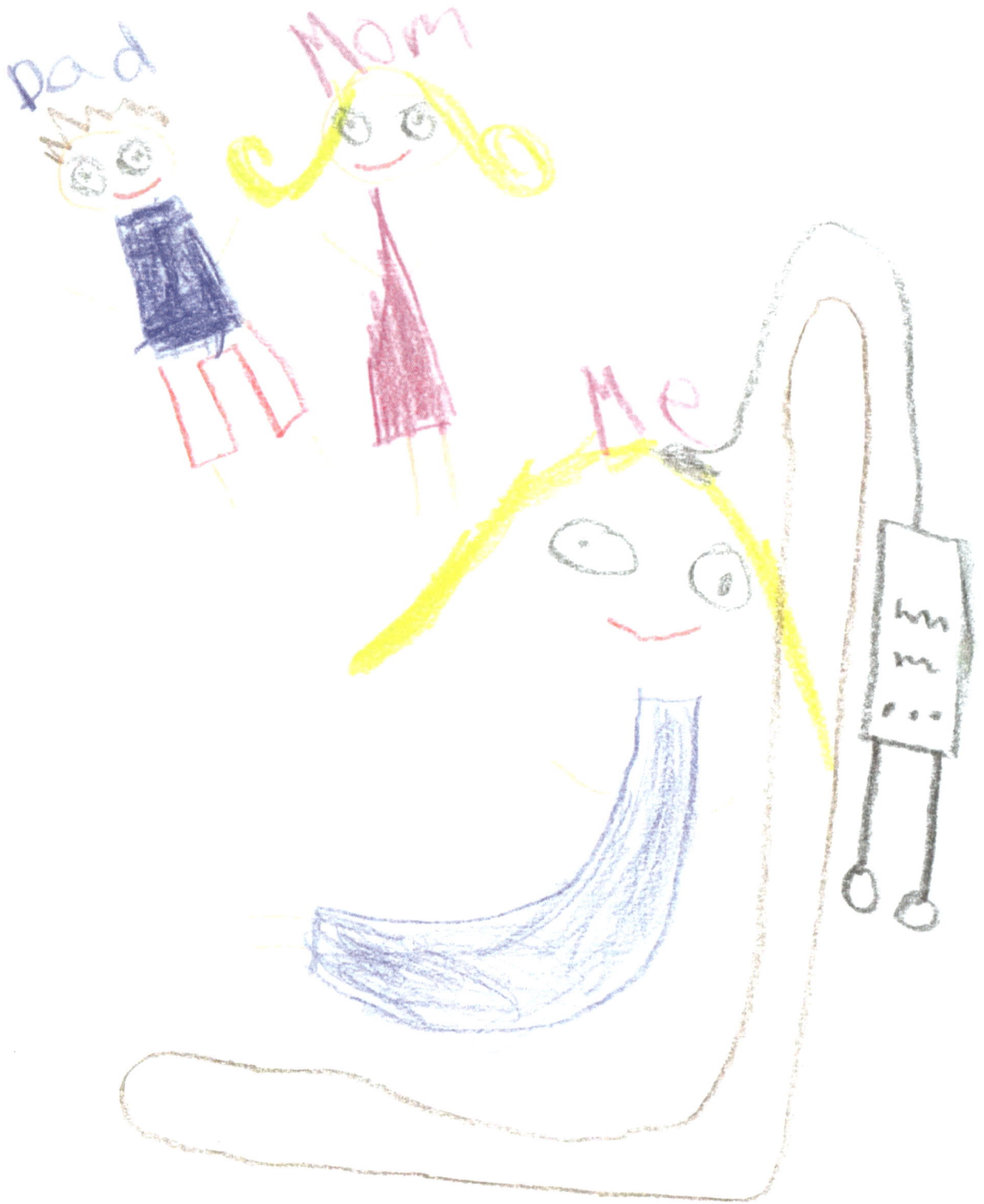

Right after the surgery, Mom and Dad came to see me in my room. I was happy to have them with me.

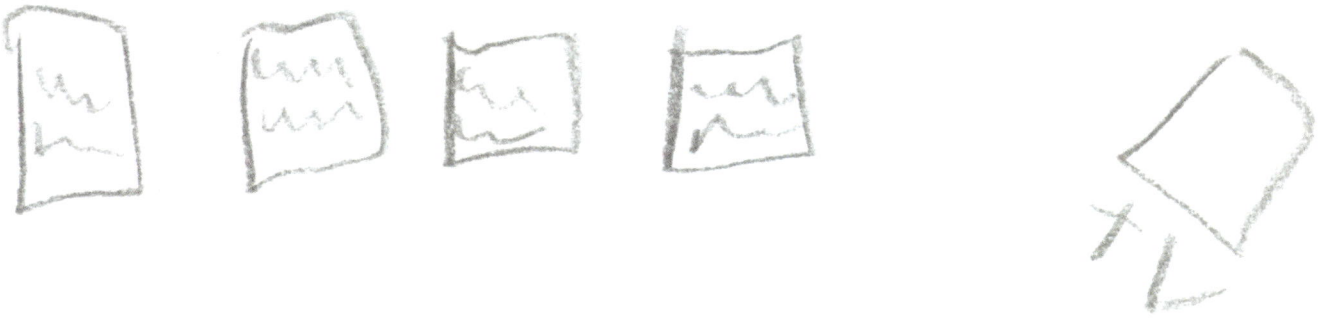

I spent a lot of time in my room resting, watching TV and playing games.

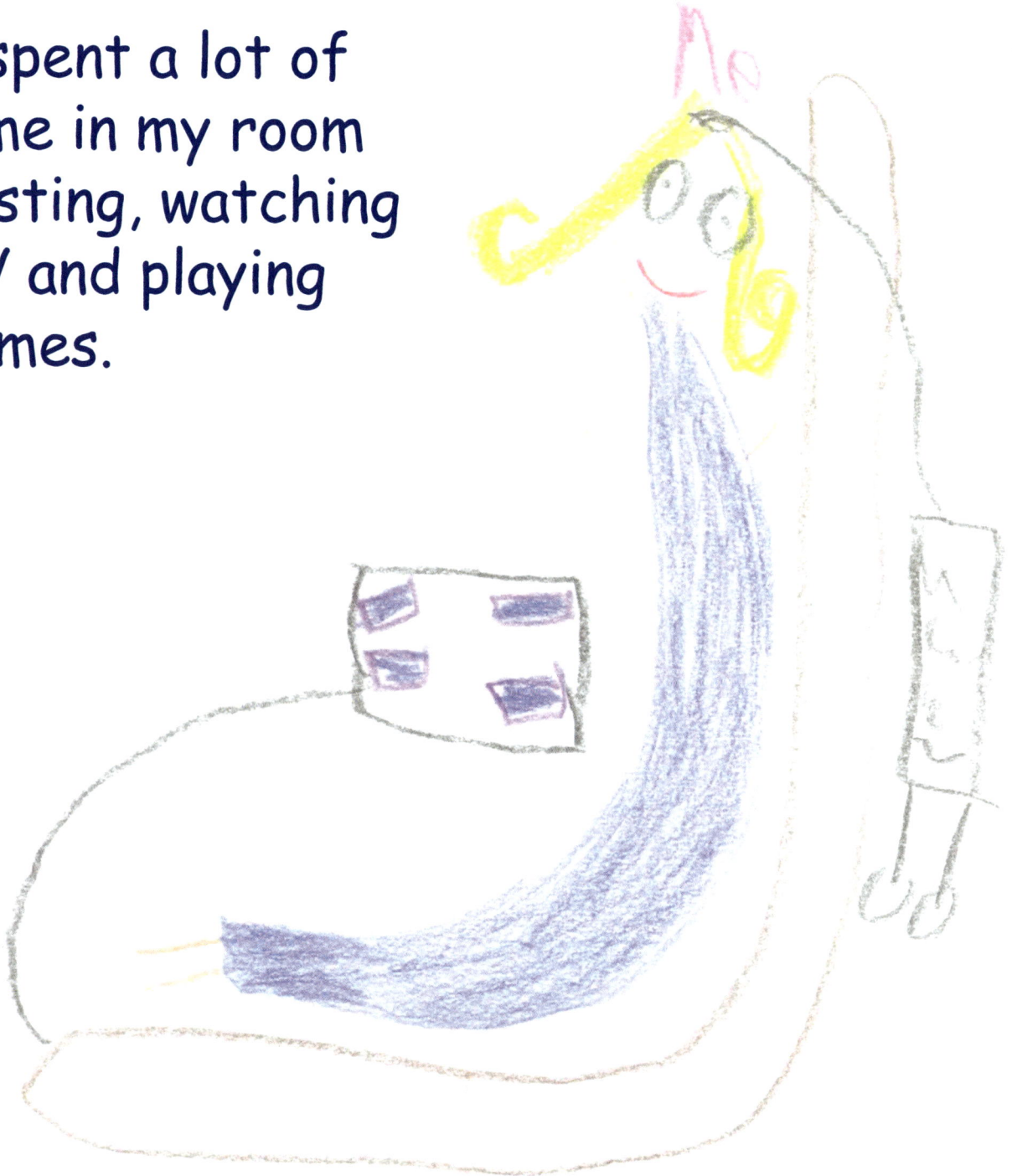

I had a lot of visitors. Sometimes I growled, sometimes I smiled, and sometimes I wanted to be alone for a while.

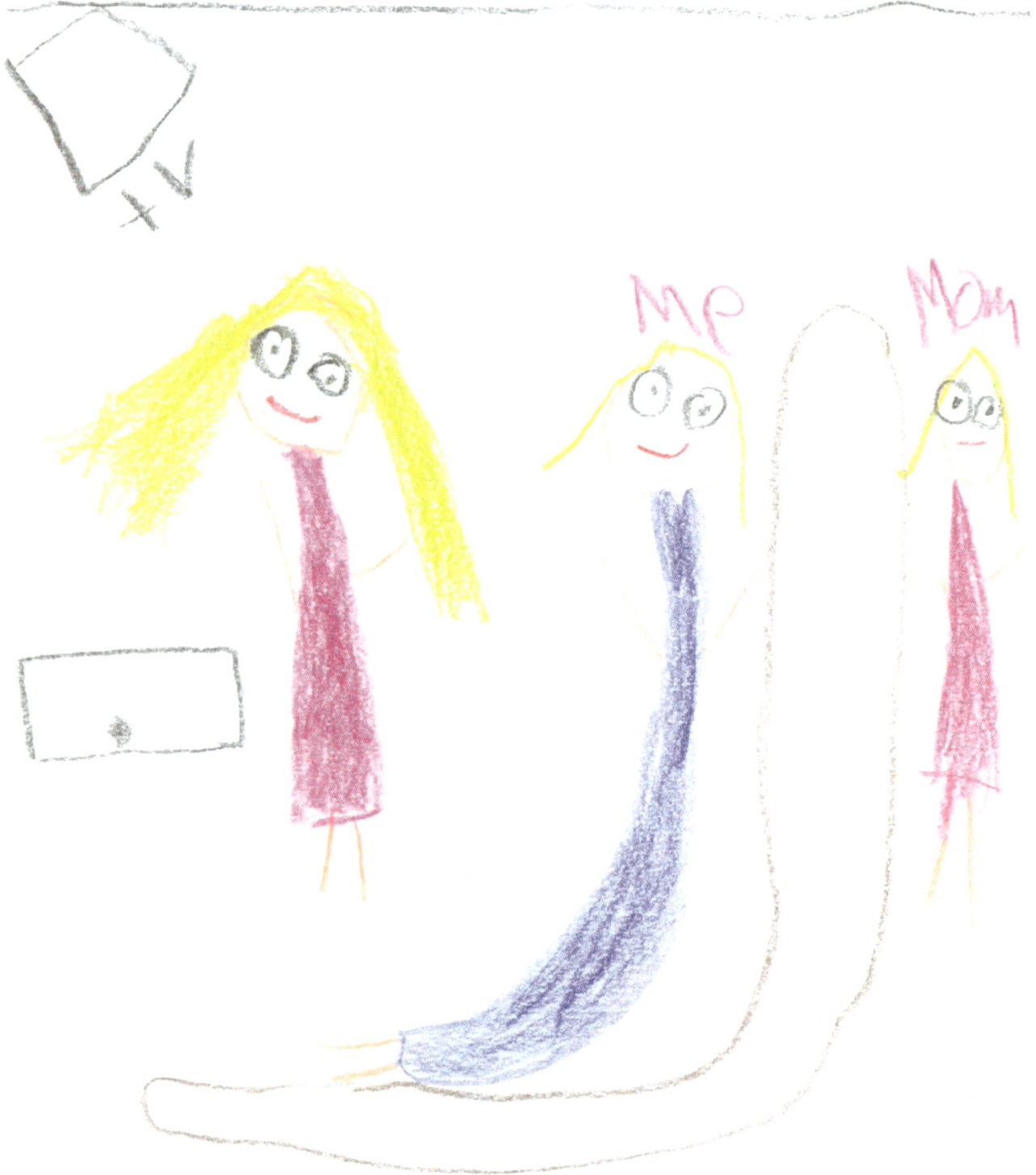

My grandma came up
with the idea of having
"Team Stacia"
for people to show their
support. We all wore
pink bracelets with
Team Stacia
written on them.

I had to have chemotherapy and radiation. The doctor put in a port where I could have my chemo done and blood drawn to make sure my blood levels were high enough to have treatment.

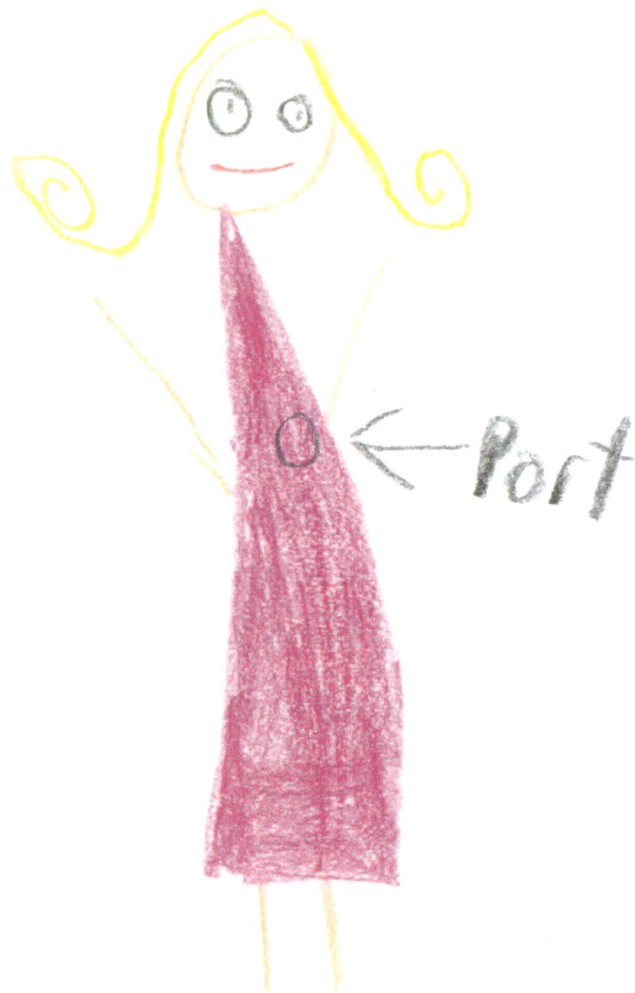

I had "sleepy cream" put on the port to numb it so I would not feel any pokes from the needle.

After my surgery, I was wobbly when I walked.

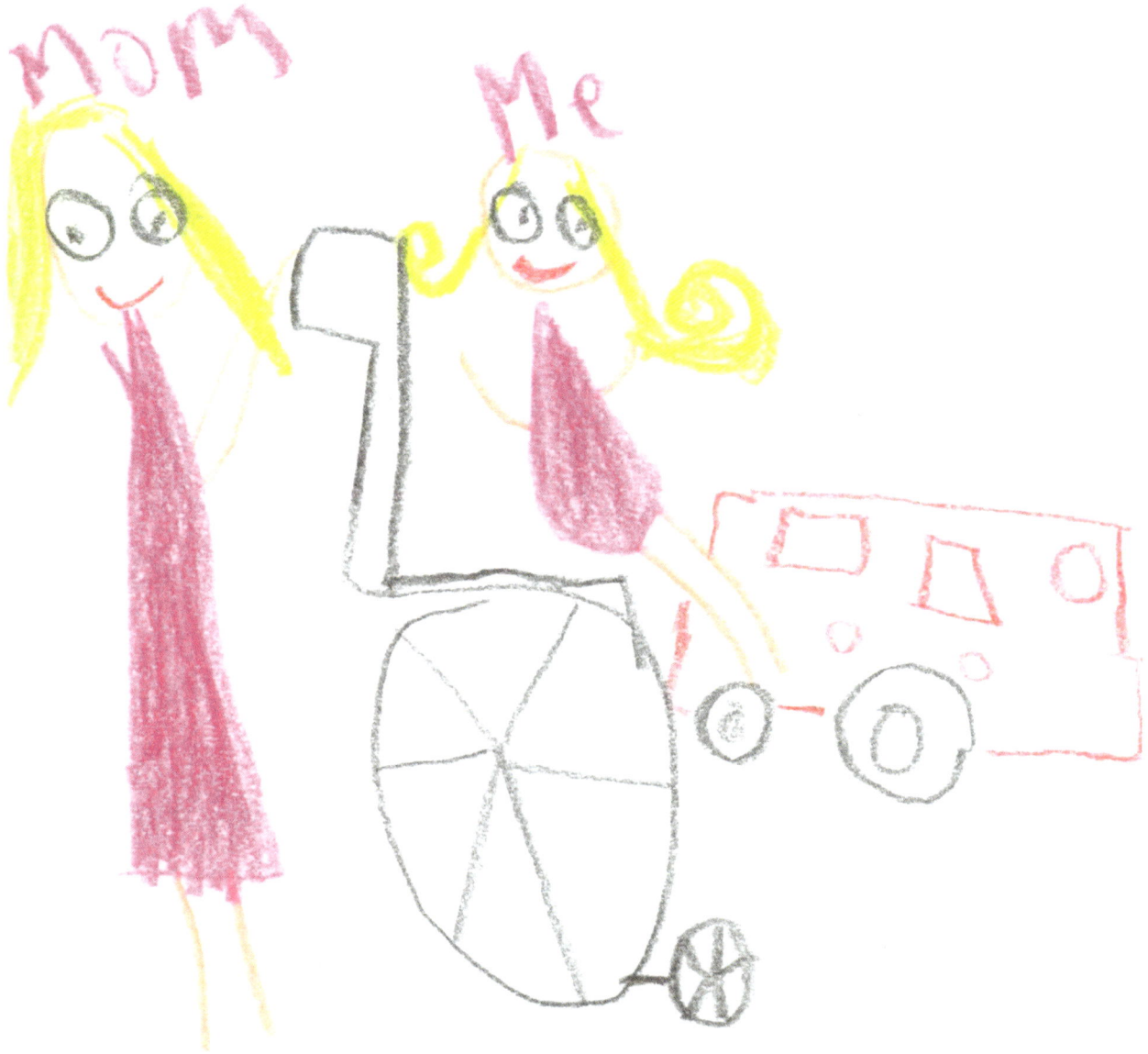

Before I was able to go home, I had to be able to walk by myself and be steady. After almost five weeks, I got to go home.

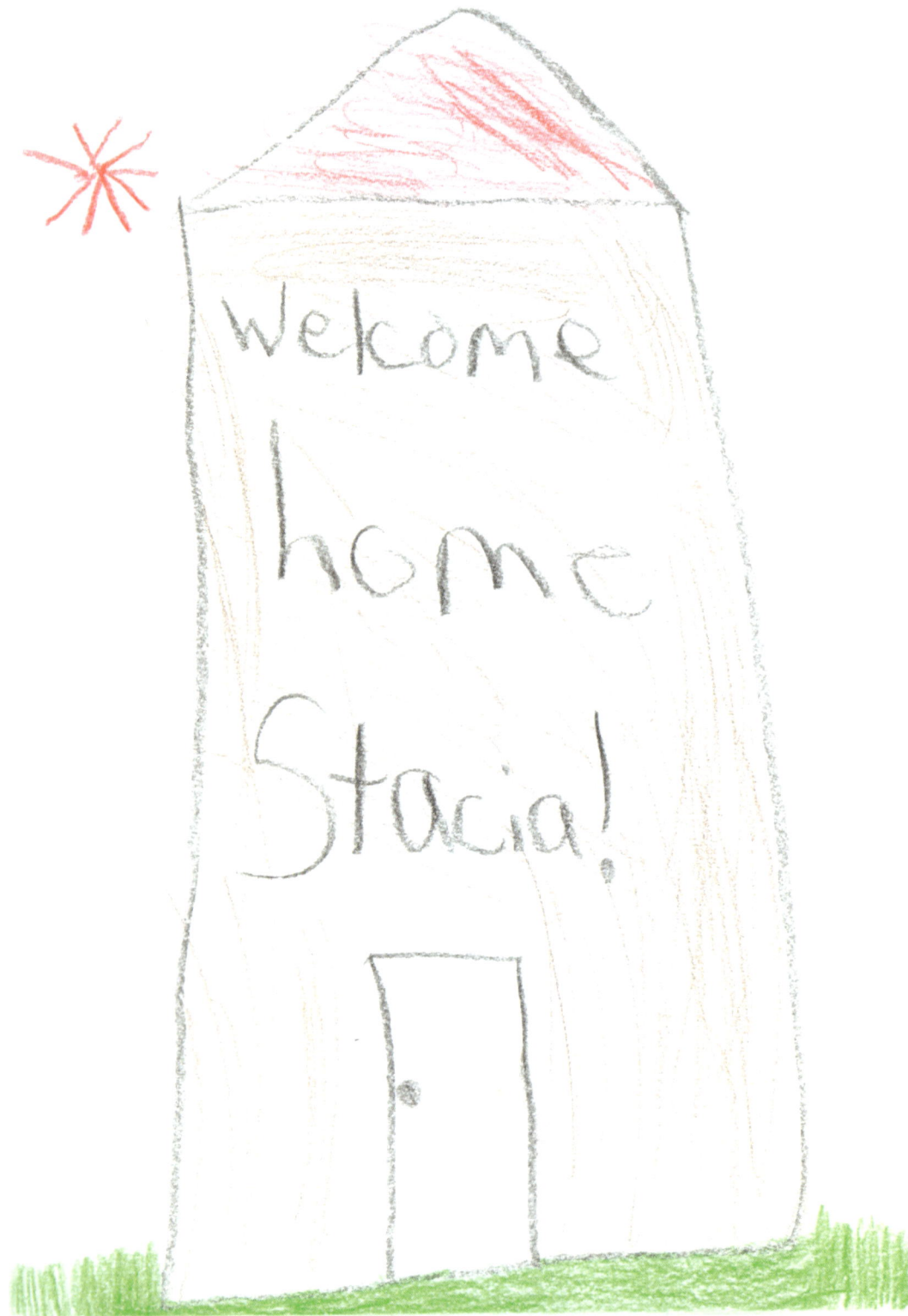

I was very glad to be home! I had to
rest and get strong so I could have
radiation and chemo.

One week later, I started six weeks of radiation, which was like rays or beams pointed where my tumor had been. Sometimes I had both radiation and chemotherapy.

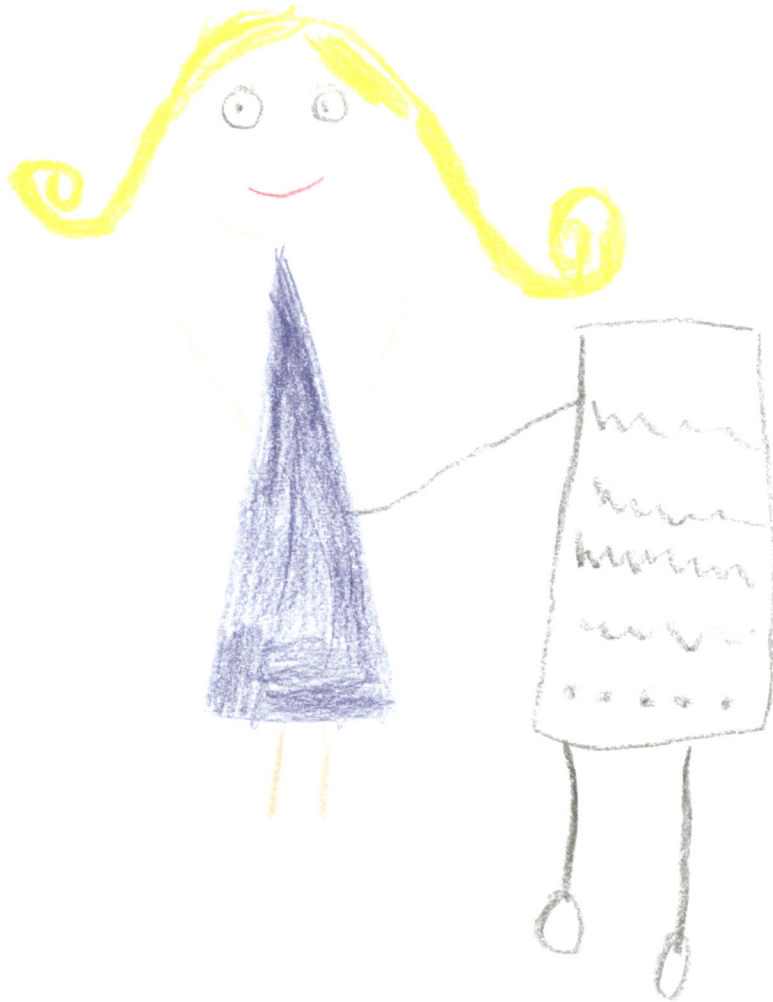

Chemo was medicine used to make sure my cancer was gone and did not come back. The radiation and chemo made me lose all of my hair.

When I had chemo, I had to stay in the hospital. I ate a lot of salmon, rice with soy sauce, asparagus and pizza.

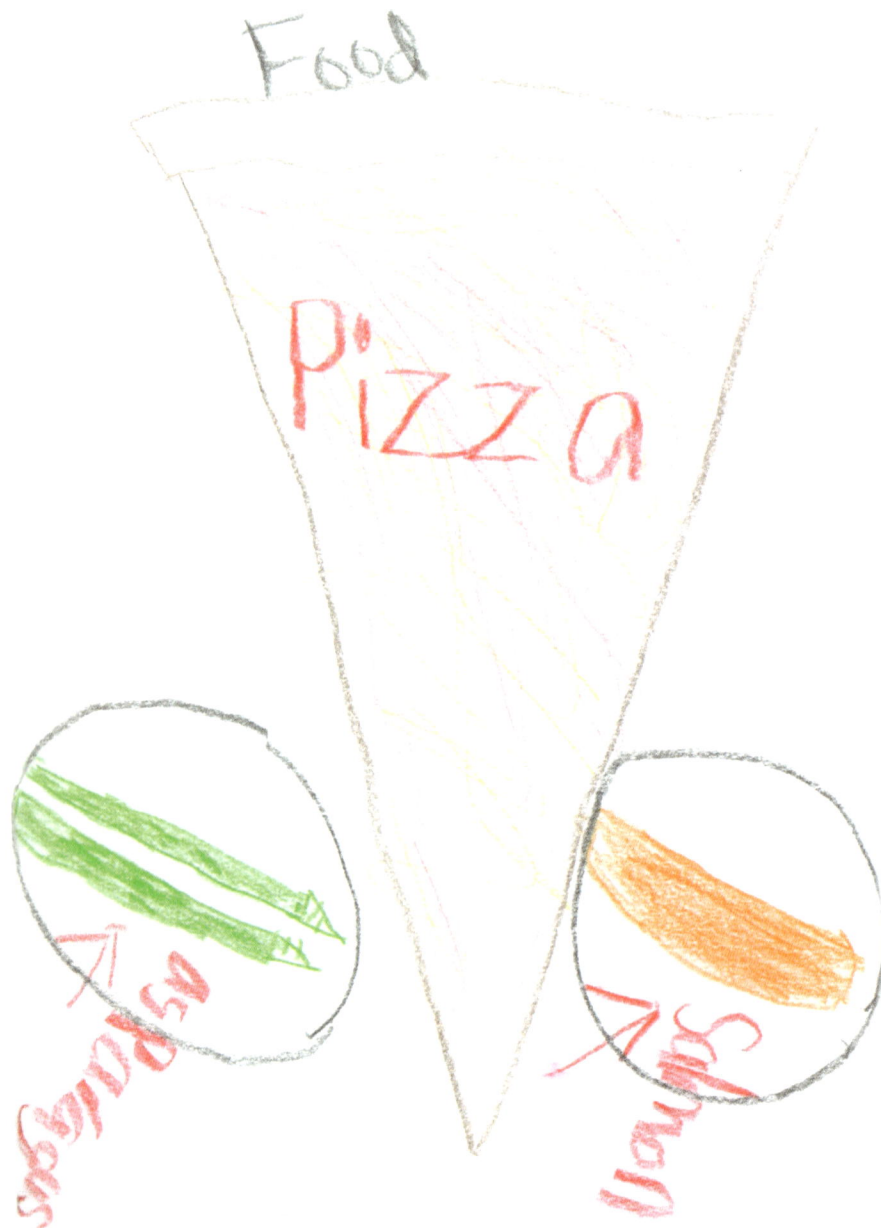

Sometimes I would get constipated, so I took other medicine to make my poop soft.

Playroom

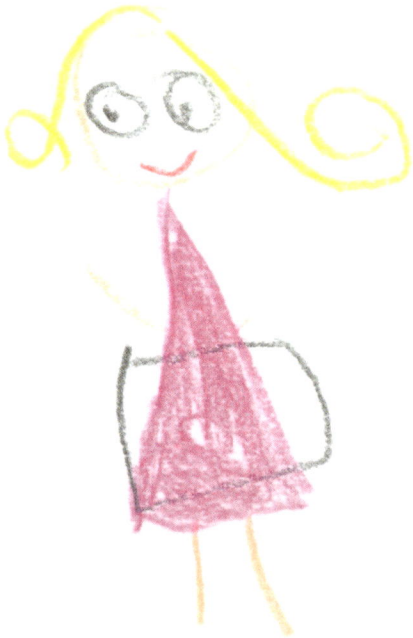

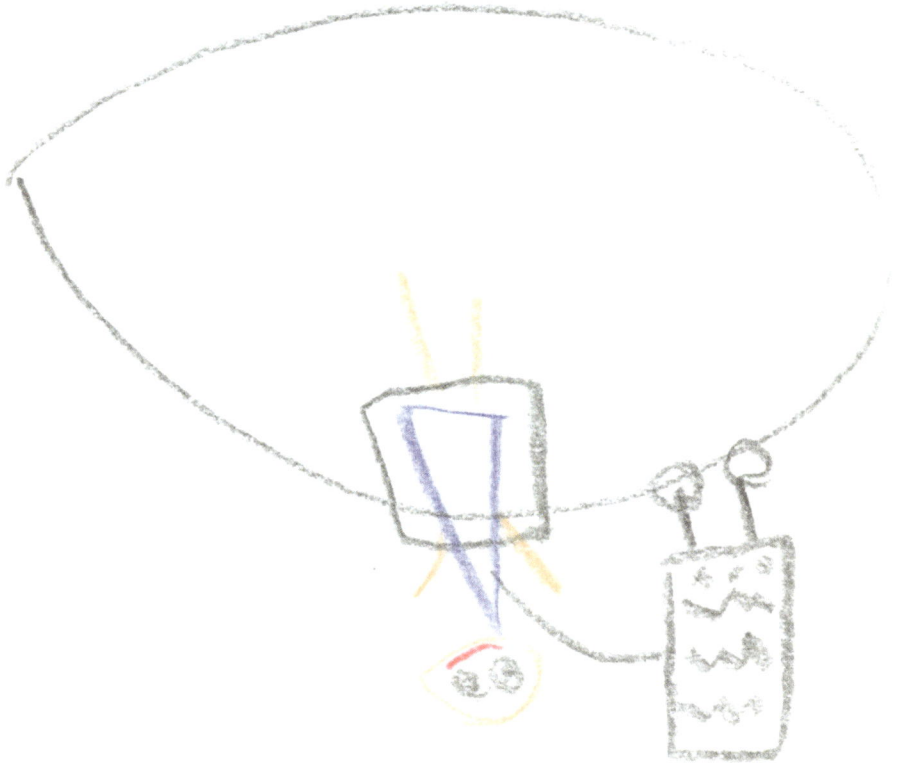

I also got to do crafts in the playroom. I had a lot of fun there. I also worked with a physical therapist to help me get stronger and a counselor to help me face my fears.

Sometimes when I tried to sleep, I had to go to the bathroom or a nurse would come in to check on my pole which held my chemo. And sometimes my pole would beep during the night.

Beep! Beep! Beep!

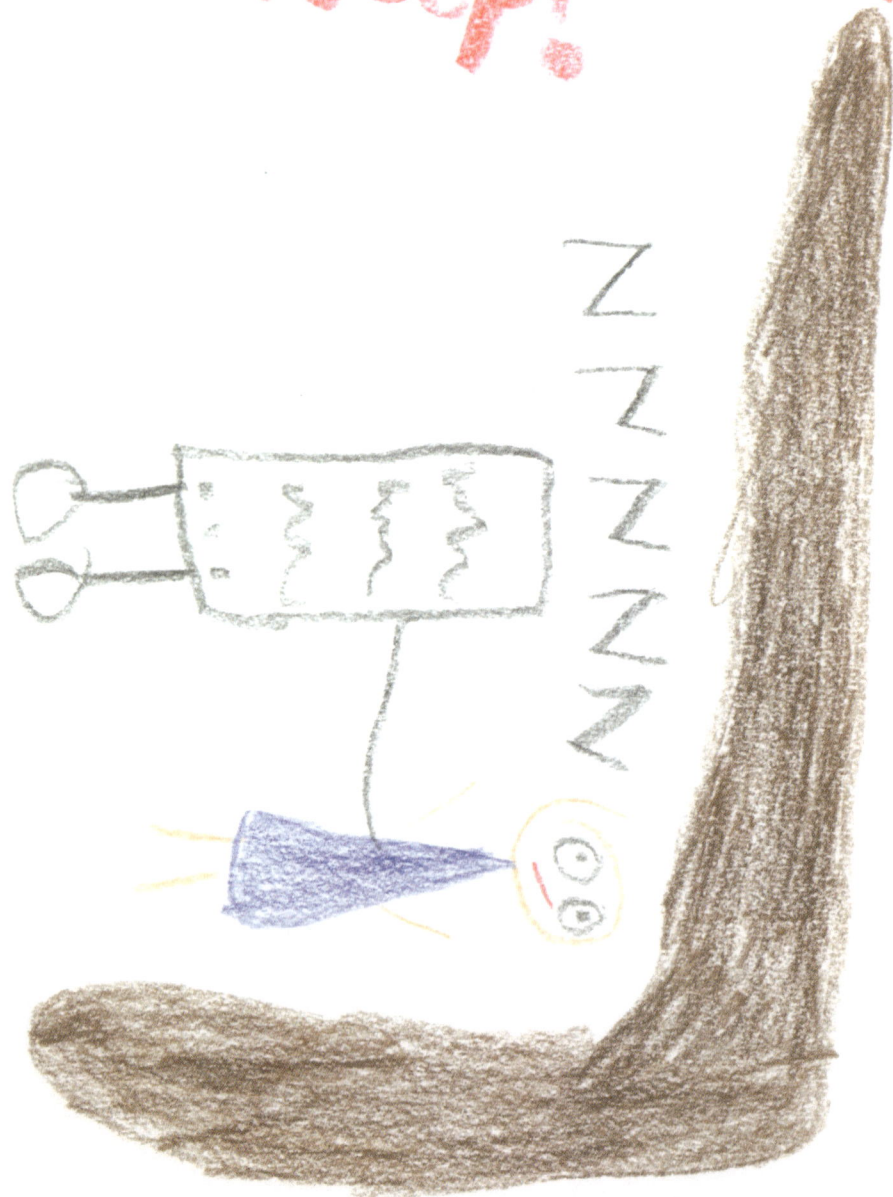

I had 14 months of chemotherapy and radiation from 2010 to 2011...

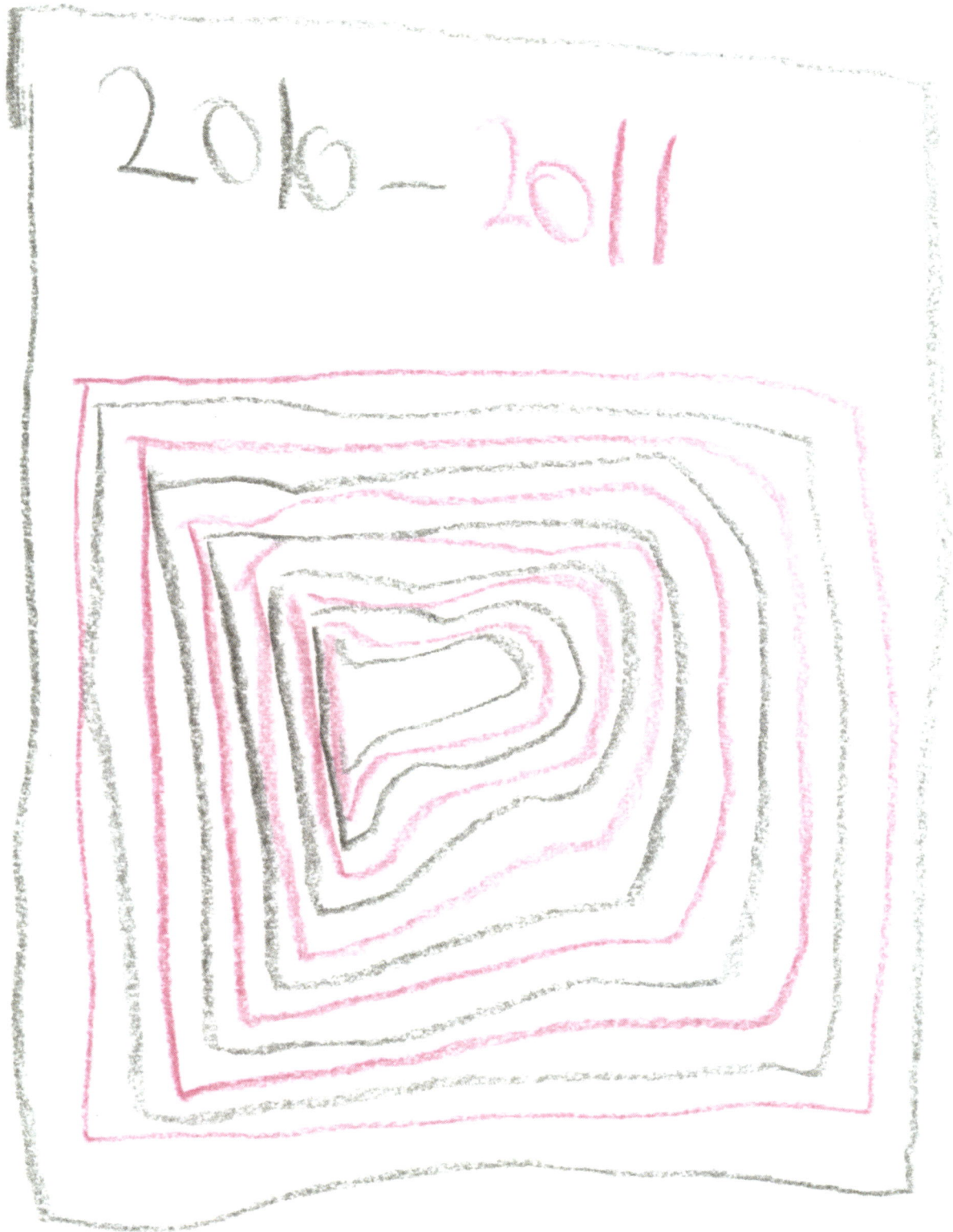

And then I was
DONE
with treatment
and had
NO
MO
CHEMO!

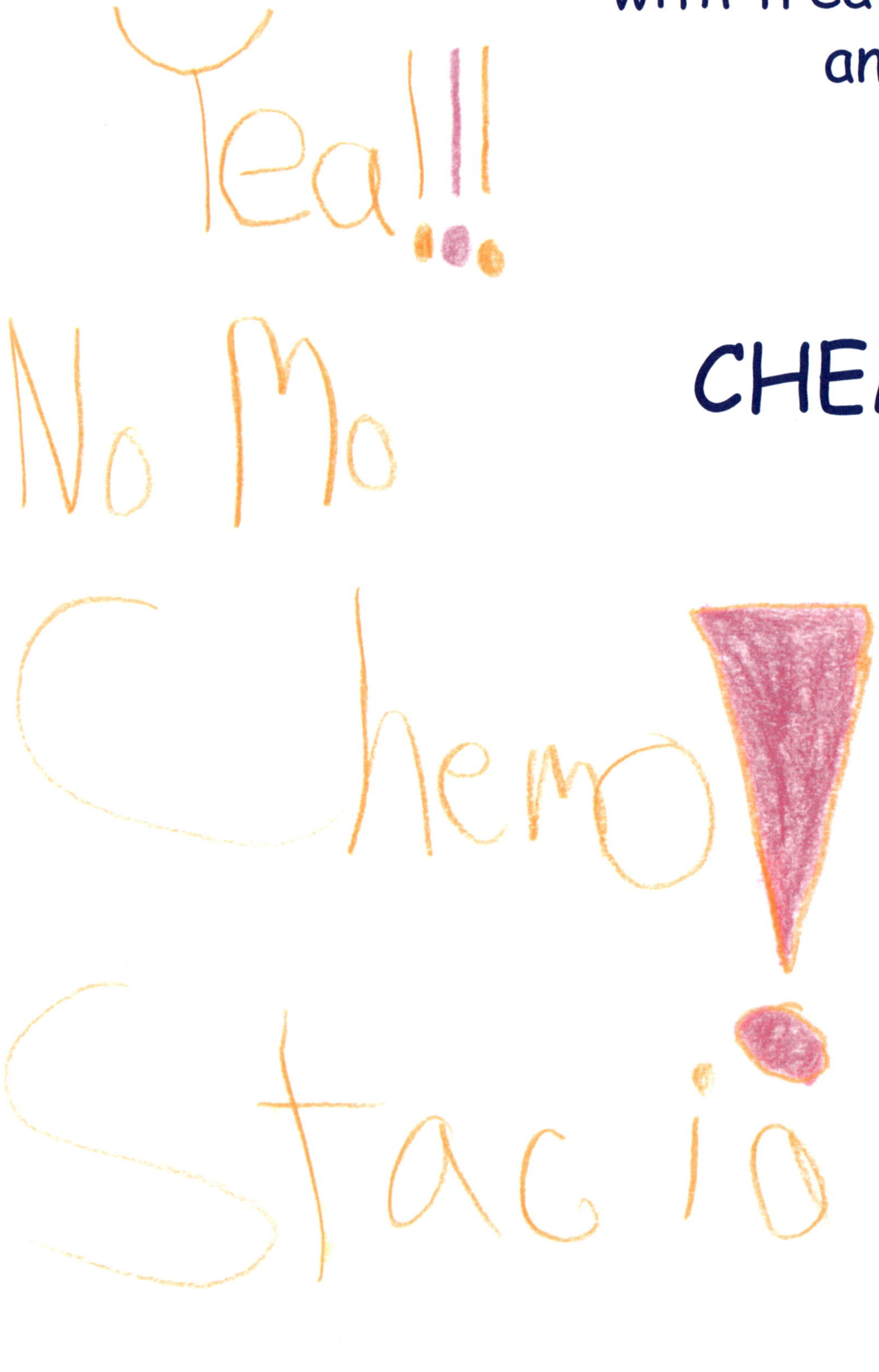

Yea!!!
No Mo
Chemo!
Stacia

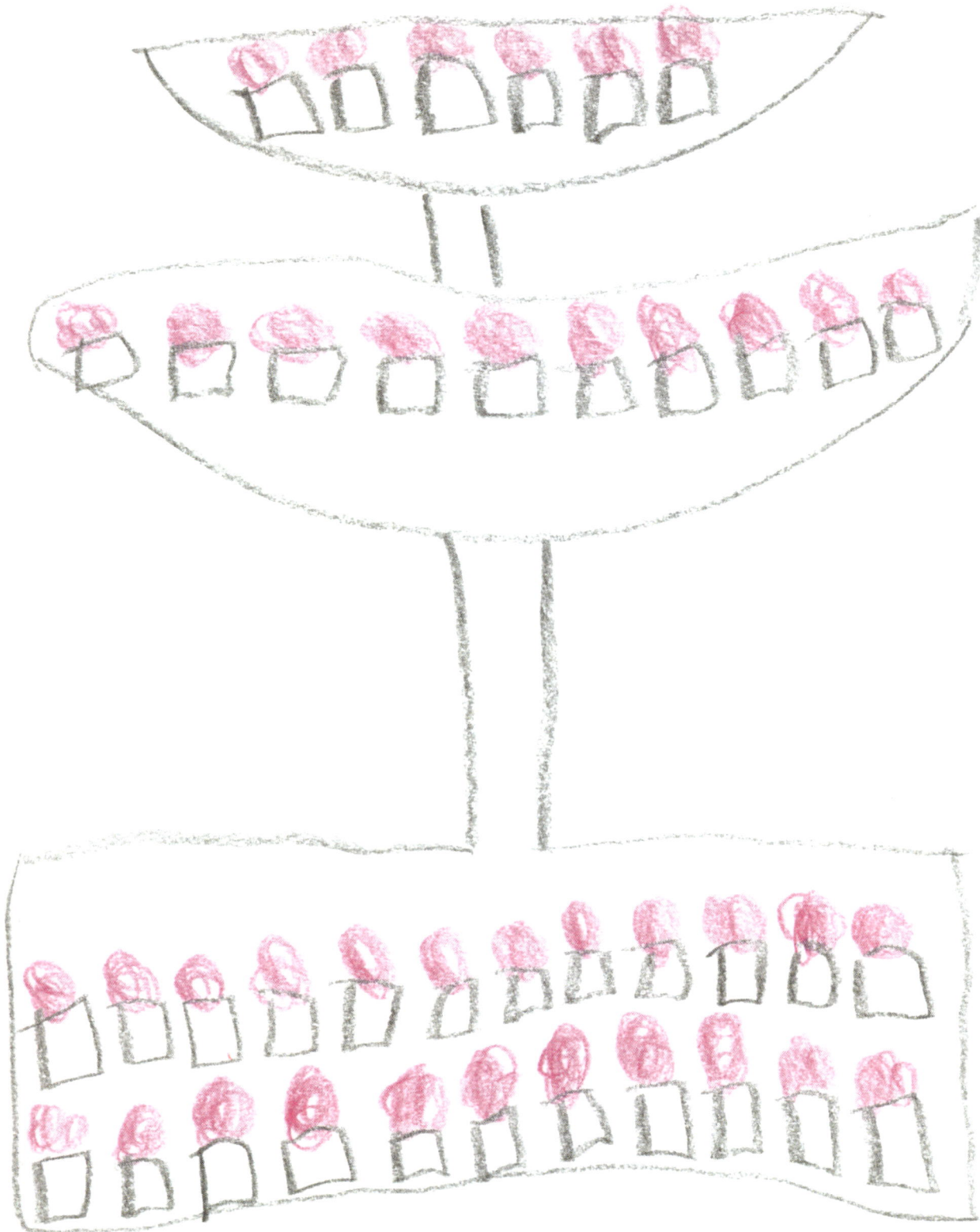

We had a party with a LOT
of PINK cupcakes!

At the party, we had a journal for everybody to sign because I made it through the treatment.

And I am glad to be done, too!

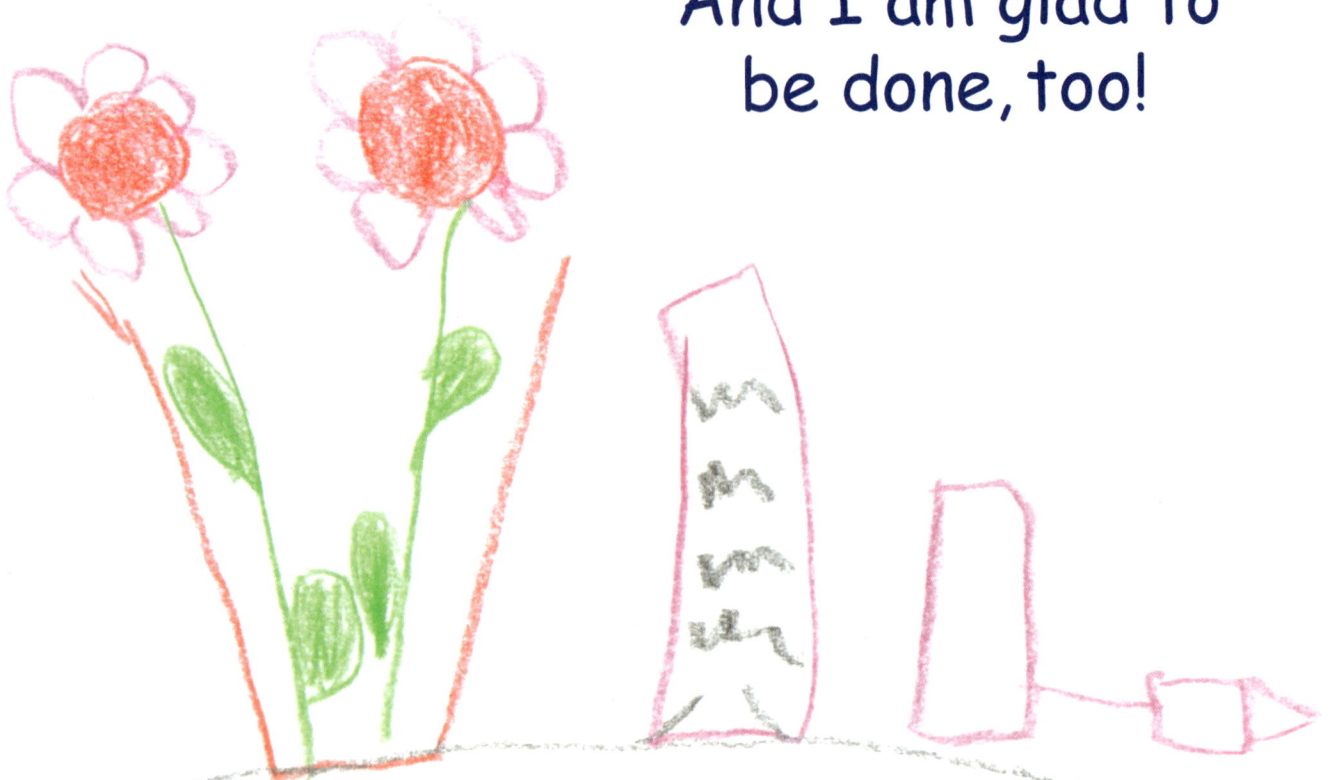

THE END